Low Carb Diet:
Easy Guide How To Lose 10 Pounds in 10 Days

Table of Content

Low Carb Diet:..1
Before we start, what is fat anyway?.....................................4
Chapter 1 – High Protein Low Carb 8
Chapter 2 – What's this going to do to my body? 13
Chapter 3 – Through the ages – Why does this work?........15
Chapter 4 – But I heard low fat diets are the way to go… 18
Chapter 5 – Myths. 20
Chapter 6 – High Fat, Low Carbohydrate Slow Cooker Chicken Recipes .23
    Buffalo Chicken 24
    Jerk Chicken..25
    Thai Green Curry Chicken..27
Chapter 7 – High Fat, Low Carbohydrate Turkey Recipes......29
    Turkey Herb Roast..29
    Turkey Mercedes..30
    Navy Style Turkey...31
    Flavorful Turkey 32
Chapter 8 – High Fat, Low Carbohydrate Beef Recipes 34
    Beef Pot Roast I..34
    Mexican Style Meat..35
    Beef Pot Roast II 37
    Roast Beef...38
Chapter 9 – High Fat, Low Carbohydrate Pork Recipes 39
    Asian Style Ribs..39
    Spicy Green Chili Pork 40

Lancaster County Pork and Sauerkraut 41
Pork Roast with Sauerkraut and Kielbasa 42
Conclusion 44

Before we start, what is fat anyway?

This is a vital question that every physique-minded individual needs to have a clear perspective on. Fat is an essential part of the body, and often the end-result of metabolizing food that provides more energy than what your body actually has spent. Let's look at fat and what's actually going on in a simple, scientific sense.

Where does fat go when you burn it off?

This is a really elementary question that everyone should know the answer to, but due to all the hype and theories and products that are being sold to us in modern society, there is a vested interest in keeping this information from you-- and that's why you probably have to guess right now.

No. You don't pass it in your bowel movements. Your bowel movements will pass non-digestible materials like fiber, and also bacteria that exist in your digestive track. There's also water in your bowl movements, and while it is an area of weight-loss and health to consider; it is not where your fat goes when you burn it off.

And no. (haha) fat isn't converted into 'pure energy'-- that only happens in thermonuclear reactions. Your body is a massively complex chemical reaction. All that's happening here is the breaking and forming of chemical bonds; no matter is converted into energy. Or at least we hope not!

The chemical formula for fat is C_{55}, H_{104}, O_6. It's a handy molecule that your body can both easily pack together from the carbon, hydrogen, and oxygen that's present in your body, and it's also really easy for your body to snag a hold of a fat-molecule, break it open and fuel some cellular respiration with.

Cellular respiration is... in essence, the act of taking an O2 oxygen molecule, breaking it apart, then letting both of those oxygen atoms bond to a carbon atom to be whisked away in the blood-stream away from a working cell. Cells take oxygen and make carbon dioxide.

So, if you'll notice, the formula for fat can make the two primary things you know your exhale-breath is made up of. Carbon dioxide and water vapor. By weight, it's about 85% carbon dioxide when fat is metabolized.

So you breathe it out. That's where fat goes.

For this physical reason, EVERY weight-loss program must follow three golden requirements, or else it's a complete and utter lie.

RULE 1: Eat less. You've got to intake less food. If you take in more food than you spend, you gain weight. If you take in less food than you spend, you lose weight.

RULE2 2: Move more. This is cellular respiration. You've got to have your cells make more carbon dioxide from oxygen. If you don't do this, you're not spending more food-- or 'fuel' as some enthusiasts refer to it.

RULE 3: Keep breathing. For obvious reasons, you're going to be breathing anyway to stay alive. But your respiratory system is where the outlet of your body-weight actually occurs. So you have to be mindful of your breathing.

ANY diet or advice that claims to make you lose weight that fails to meet these requirements should be met with the highest amount of skepticism. This is the basic formula for all weight-loss.

However, there are techniques for achieving results that follow these rules and optimize the whole process in such a way that makes it much easier to stay on track with your weight-loss goals.

A typical high-protein / low carb diet can make a regular person lose up to 10 pounds of 'real' weight in 10 days. Or roughly a pound a day for the first ten days, depending on how afflicted they were before hand. Obviously, if you're already hovering at a low body fat percentage, you probably won't have much fat to burn, and won't see those weight-loss goals.

But if you're someone with very low body-fat, either you are genetically blessed to have a fast metabolism (most of us aren't; a fast metabolism is a survival-liability, actually) or you're at a low body-fat percentage already through your own hard work, you probably don't need to be on a diet like the one that's going to be described here.

This diet is designed to re-tool your body's digestion system to burn fat and possibly build muscle depending on how much exercise you have. It's not a magical wand to waive over your body-- there are no shortcuts; just paths that keep you on the straight and narrow. The shortest distance between two points is a straight line, and we're going to show you one of those straight-shot destinations that you can stick with here.

For this cookbook, you will need a thorough understanding of how to measure the temperatures of different meats to know if they are finished cooking. Therefore, you will need a meat thermometer. In addition to that, it would be a good idea to have a slow cooker or crockpot in order to be able to complete these recipes. Always check the internal temperature of meat to make sure that it is finished cooking as times can vary a little.

The following is a chart of the temperatures of different types of meats in this cookbook and their done temperatures.

Chicken	180°F (82°C)
Turkey	180°F (82°C)
Beef	165°F (74°C)
Pork	180°F (82°C)

The recipes in this cookbook are specifically for a high fat, low carbohydrate diet; therefore, all the recipes will reflect this. All recipes will have a maximum of eighteen grams of carbohydrates or less.

Chapter 1 – High Protein Low Carb

What does it do and how does it work?

Well... It's a diet designed to force your body into burning fat. It accomplishes this based on a pretty well-known exploit that your body is going to go for the most easily-available source of energy that it can find. Carbohydrates are a metabolic power-house. Your body can break down complex carbohydrates into all sorts of stuff and then convert that straight into fat and store it if you don't burn it immediately-- which most people don't.

But hey, if you're a marathon athlete, or you're in an elite military training course, or you're just one of those people who has tons of trouble putting on weight, maybe you can get away with loading up on carbs and simple starches and get away with it.

For anyone else-- and for the typical person reading this, your weight-loss potential can vary somewhat, but generally this is the fastest way to lose weight over a 10-day period. A pound of body-fat can be burnt through every day with only moderate exercise if you are following strictly this diet.

-example diets

UNDER ALL PHASES OR ITERATIONS OF THESE DIETS, IT IS CRITICAL THAT YOU ABSOLUTELY MINIMIZE YOUR EXPOSURE TO ALL CARBOHYDRATES SUCH AS:

1. Bread.

2. Potatoes.

3. High Fructose Corn Syrup.

4. Rice.

5. Starches.

6. Baked goods.

7. Virtually any food-stuff item or fast food.

8. Minimize dairy

YOU SHOULD HAVE UNDER 3 OZ PER 100 POUNDS OF YOUR CURRENT BODY-WEIGHT OF THESE CARBOHYDRATES DAILY; IF YOU GO OVER YOU ARE NOT FOLLOWING THESE DIET PLANS.

<u>Carbohydrate cleanse</u>-- this is used at the beginning of a high-protein/low carb diet. It shocks the body and prepares body-fat to be burned off.

-Drink over 1 gallon of water a day

-Have only two large meals a day, with three snacks allowed every day.

-Have as much leafy greens like spinach, broccoli or lettuce as you want in your meals.

-Eat up to 20 oz. Of pork, beef, or other red meats per 100 pounds of bodyweight that you have at that time per day

-Season foods as you will; salt is not bad at this point in the diet.

-Snacks should be pairs of items of fruit, such as a single banana and an apple, or a box of raisins with a peach. Only have citrus fruits a maximum of once a day under this diet.

<u>Fat-burner</u>-- After you have done the previous diet for at least five days, switch to this diet which will squeeze weight (mostly in the form of fat and water) off of your body like ringing out a rag.

-Drink under but *up to* 1 gallon of water a day, or only to satisfy thirst. (Do NOT drink sports-drinks or sodas)

-Eat two or one meal a day of minimal size. Have four snacks a day, but make them even smaller.

-Have lean proteins in your meals. White chicken breast, egg whites (separate the yolk), tuna, or salmon. Have 16oz of these kinds of lean protein foods per 100 pounds of body-weight per day.

-Avoid sodium. Season your foods with garlic powder, cinnamon (yes, even on meats-- and make sure it's real cinnamon and not cassia)

-Snacks here should be single food-items and centered around citrus fruits or green apples. Have oranges, Clementine, raisins, or grapes. Try to pick snacks of a sour taste.

-If you absolutely get very hungry and feel you need to eat, have a glass of water and enough celery to fill you.

-Engage in exercises like swimming, jogging, or bicycling.

Muscle-enhancer-- For some of you, you may be interested in burning fat but also gaining muscle. The above diets will burn fat but make you lose weight. It's possible to burn fats while being weight-neutral or actually gaining weight, but only gaining muscle weight.

-Eat three meals a day with snacks. The frequency of the snacks should be 1 hour after you notice that you are feeling hungry, if the meal is not under an hour away.

-Have small sources of protein such as cans of tuna, or pouches of almonds. When you are feeling hungry, have a handful of nuts or a can of fish and see how you feel in an hour before having more.

-Diversify your protein-sources. Have steak, salmon, chicken, vineson, pork, pento beans, and keenwa-- but keep changing the protein-source with maybe two common lean proteins such as chicken breast and egg-whites.

-Allow one carbohydrate: Sweet potatoes. And have no more than 2 sweet potatoes a day. Do not have any other kind of potato.

-Have high-fiber foods like sunflower or flax seeds-- or even triscuits if you're in an absolute pinch.

-Snack on dried prunes, raisins, leafy greens, and jerky.

-Eat according to hunger, but slowly, and stop as soon as you feel the food 'hit you.' You'll want to be close to calorie-neutral.

-You should experience at least two bowel movements a day under this; if you are not, then you need to take in more fiber and dried prunes.

-Engage in exercises such as weight-lifting if you are trying to add muscle mass, or light weight resistance training if you are trying to tone muscle. Continue with cardio-exercises such as jogging, cycling, or swimming.

These are just a few sources of protein that you may be able to incorporate into your diet pretty easily. And avoid carbohydrates as much as possible since they're 'sticky' foods.

If you stick with this and exercise, you can lose up to 1 pound a day for the first 10 days!

Chapter 2 – What's this going to do to my body?

The short answer is it just makes your body lose fat because you're cutting out the kind of stuff that it uses to make fat easily-- and you're replacing it with proteins which are much more difficult for your body to make fat with.

That doesn't mean that this is some sort of absolute panacea to weight-loss. If you don't exercise at all and you hork down bacon all day of course you're going to be technically following our guidelines, but you're also going to gain weight and possibly even have a heart-attack. So what kinds of exercises are recommended with this diet?

Well... That depends on what your goals are. And also what kinds of proteins you are taking in. If you're taking in red meats, you may be more apt to build bulky muscle on a diet like that, so weight-training with the heaviest weights you can safely manage might be a good option to quickly build muscle mass while losing fat-- almost as if you were converting your fat into muscle. If you go this route, you're going to probably want to actually gain weight on this kind of diet, which means you're going to have to intake more calories than you spend. But again you'll still be losing fat content even though you're at a positive-sum gain in overall weight because of the muscle mass you're going to be packing on.

But you can also lean down quite a bit on a diet like this too. In fact, most professional body builders eat like this to get their body-fat percentages down very very low, which makes for visible muscles.

So you may want to go with lean proteins like almonds and white meats like chicken breast and do a considerable amount of cardio. Cardio is also regarded as the most enjoyable exercise that athletes prefer to do since it's so natural for the body to be in motion for long periods of time.

Intense cardio exercises on lean-proteins will probably cut straight into your body fat percentage, and the proteins will probably help your body resist the urge to begin feeding on its own muscle mass as an energy source-- especially if you're running long-term caloric deficits, which you should be if you're trying to cut down on your body-fat percentage.

If you already have bulky muscles, you can shred them up on this kind of diet as well. Shredding is the process of losing weight, but gaining muscular definition. You'll run very gentle caloric deficits while doing light or middle-weight exercises with very high repetition. This will cut into your body fat and squeeze into your muscles. It'll also have a perceived effect of tightening your skin.

All of these things are achievable because you're training your body to burn protein as fuel rather than relying on simple starches and carbohydrates. It's like forcing your body into over-drive and making it work much harder on a cellular level. It will increase your metabolism, but it's also something that you need to keep in check; while some people do use these diets for extended periods of time, there have been some health risks that have been pointed out about the high-protein low-carb diet.

Mainly critics of this diet state that this diet can be linked to heart-problems and other organ-based oddities-- and they may be right! So if you're on a diet like this, generally keep it to three months, and only stay on a diet like this if you're actually pushing for some sort of goal that is related to your exercise routine. Don't do this just because you think you're going to automatically lose weight; this isn't exactly the most natural diet in the world, so be in control of what's going on, and more importantly be aware of any apparent changes in your body.

The most stable diet in the world is the well-rounded diet, which eats a wide variety of things from a diverse range of sources and food groups. This high-protein low-carb diet is much more specific to burning off fat and packing on or toning muscle. So keep that in mind while you're on this kind of diet.

Chapter 3 – Through the ages – Why does this work?

Okay so you remember how we just said that this isn't the most natural diet in the world? Well... we probably should have said it's not the most 'typical' diet in the world. As in the modern world.

As it turns out... How do you think humans-- for the most part-- ate over the ages? Do you think we had access to High Fructose Corn Syrup (HFCS) while we were running away from chimpanzees at the beginning of our species' lives? Heck no. So how do you think we ate?

There wasn't Starbucks back in those days. And we also know through fossil records that we did have very large brains early on in our species' history. Those big brains require a lot of very dense calories. IE proteins. More specifically... animal proteins. So we were eating animals. And we would eat meat pretty regularly, as fossil records indicate.

So, you have to have access to eating other animals in order to get the calorie densities that you need to have and sustain in order to evolve intelligence as a species. So basically it's kind of like a chicken and the egg thing with us, our intelligence, and our ability to successfully eat protein from animals.

We know we could not have used our intelligence to hunt animals all along, because we know that we need to hunt other animals for a very, very long period of time before we even get the ability to sustain these calorie-demanding brains of ours.

It turns out that we humans are freakishly good at two things aside from our intelligence. Guess what they are.

Drumroll please?

The first one is... SWEATING! I know. Anticlimactic, right? But we're actually one of the only animals who can breathe, cool ourselves (sweat) and run all at the same time. In comparison, a horse can do any two of those three...

The second one is... THROWING! That's more clever, isn't it? But it's not something you think about. But we are spooky-good at throwing. In fact, you can blind-fold your average human being, give them a ball, then throw some keys in the air and we can get kind of close to actually hitting the keys with the ball while the keys are in air! The next closest thing to that in the animal kingdom is the fact that chimps will sometimes sling poo side-handed.

So for most of our evolutionary history, we were chasing after animals-- like deer-- in groups, throwing things at it. We would do this for about four or five hours at a time, and as long as we kept the poor thing in motion for those four or five hours, the beast would fall over DEAD from heat exhaustion. Score. We got us some meat.

We would also use our frontally-aligned visual receptors (eyes) to pick out a little critter some ways off, and then we'd hurl a heavy-ish object at it and hopefully kill it that way. Score. We got more meat that way.

Another interesting theory about our evolution is that ... have you noticed how we're naked and our chimp-brethren are all furry?

Some biologists think that this is because we might've spent much more time in and around the water than our ape-cousins. It would make sense; body-hair definitely resists the flow of water quite a lot.

And we probably did eat a good amount of fish. Our technique for hunting fish probably involved just corralling them into spots where they were easier to poke or grab or splash up on shore.

It's a good theory but there's less concrete evidence on this one.

So all through our history, we've always ate more meat than we have carbohydrates; it would make sense for our bodies to have adapted to function under this ancient kind of diet much more than our modern, carbohydrate-laden diets.

We also used to move around quite a bit; we were agrarian for the longest period of our evolutionary history. We'd sort of roam from one place to another scattering useful seeds of berries and nuts that we'd gather and eat.

So there you have it; meat, berries, and nuts. That's what we've been eating for most of our evolutionary histories. And there are many diets-- like the paleo diet-- that try to underscore this. And they work. People are healthy under regiments of much more exercise, proteins, and hardly any carbohydrates if any at all.

Incidentally, the modern person today has much more fat stored on their bodies than the early humans did. So following the behavioral patterns of what are essentially 'cave-men' can and will burn fat off of your body as fast as safely possible.

These are primarily eating meats nuts and berries, as well as increasing your aerobic exercises. Do this, and the fat will melt away from your body in a short amount of time.

Chapter 4 – But I heard low fat diets are the way to go...

That's a common misconception. Just because you are eating fat doesn't mean that it's going to be turned into fat-- your body doesn't work like that. You don't intake animal fat in your stomach and that somehow gets transported as-is to your love handles.

Every kind of food gets broken down in to really, really small components and dispersed throughout the blood-stream, where these components are assembled by cells based on their availability in the blood-stream, and the biological activity of these cells.

So no; eating a gram of fat doesn't mean that you're going to necessarily gain a gram of fat-- in fact, you'll never be able to gain fat from fat at a 100% efficiency rate. So if you take a gram of fat in, the very most you can gain from it will be less than one gram of fat.

Low-fat diets are just appealing to peoples' ignorance. They don't actually mean you're going to lose fat on your body.

By comparison the high protein low carb diet is a scientific fact. It is effective at cutting down the fat content of your body.

The real killer of any diet is the carbohydrate. Your body is very effective at turning those into fats and clogging up your arteries with things like butters and sugars and fatty acids. You need to be very careful of the carbohydrate. The protein, by comparison is much less threatening than the carbohdydrate. It can pretty much be used for just one of two things.

It can be burned for energy. And it can be used for cellular structures like muscle. Else it tends to pass right through you, provided that your body isn't in starvation mode and you're not moving at all.

Sadly most nutritionists still go the easy route and recommend what people want to hear-- which is a 'low fat' diet. But have you noticed how-- due to the low fat diet's massive popularity-- pretty much all the foods in the grocery stores 'contain no fat!'?

Are there still fat people? Yes. Yes people are still generally way more out of shape than they ever should be. And they're eating fatless foods. So there's your observable proof that your body-fat comes from sources other than intaking animal fat.

Avocados have a high fat content-- and they may be the healthiest food on this planet! Eat your avocados! They're great for you, even if they're a little calorie dense-- and ESPECIALLY if they're calorie dense!

We'll get to this in the next chapter. There's a lot of myths surrounding this topic that we're going to have to debunk in order to give you the clearest perspective on how to lose weight and live a healthy lifestyle.

According to the available science though, of all the diets that you can safely go on, the high-protein low-carb diet is the only one that is scientifically proven to burn fat at a fast and yet safe rate. It's simple science; really.

Chapter 5 – Myths.

There are a great deal of myths surrounding the topic of weight-loss. Everyone knows this. Marketing hype is mostly to blame for this, since unfortunately most of commerce is dependent on peoples' ignorance.

Here's the low-down on some of the worst myths; and we've already covered the "fat free" diets that can make you fat in the last chapter.

Biggest myth: Calories, it's all in the calories

Yes and no-- but mostly no. Calories are a measure of the chemical energy that's stored in a food. WEIGHT loss is about... well... losing weight; not energy. So something being very calorie dense just means that if you don't spend the energy that's stored in the food, it'll probably turn into fat.

Some of the best foods available for your body are remarkably calorie-dense. Avocados being a prime example. Eat avocados and get considerable amounts of cardio on a daily basis and you'll be fine. The smaller the mass of the food-intake, and the more energy you actually spend throughout the day is what you need to be considering when you look at losing weight. It's that balance that determines weight loss.

It's also why the paleo diet is so effective at making people lose weight.

Second biggest myth: You can improve your physique without effort.

There are a kajillion claims that you can lose weight seemingly by just taking some pill or refraining from doing some thing. For most concerns, you can regard the pills as false claims, and also consider how all of the thing you'd have to refrain from doing are things that we instinctively do, like eating at a calorie-surplus-- so it'll require effort to actually not do them.

Third biggest myth: The fat free diet.

We've already explained this, but you can be totally fat-free on your intake, and if you have a calorie surplus for the day, your body is going to make and store some fat; there's no way around that. Especially if you're intaking carbohydrates.

Fourth biggest myth: Ab workouts and visible abs.

No. Just no. You can do crunches all you want and build the prettiest abdominal muscles ever, but if they're buried under a layer of fat, they're going to never be seen. Six-packs are a feature of low body-fat; and much less a feature of doing ab exercises.

Some body-builders don't even do or recommend abdominal-only exercises. This is primarily because your abdominals are used in... well... pretty much everything. They're a stabilizing muscle group. So if you work these out first before you go weight-lifting, you're going to increase your chances of tweaking a muscle and seriously hurting yourself.

Fifth biggest myth: "Genetics"

Yes. Genetics to play a part in your body. But that part that they do play is vastly inferior to the influence your personal lifestyle choices that you take. And genetics will never trump physics. Remember the three bare-minimum golden rules of weight loss: Eat less, move more, keep breathing.

Genetics can't ruin this. Another thing worth mentioning is that nobody is beautiful by default (at least not for men)-- every good body takes effort, and consistency over the long term. So genetics can somewhat bless you, and somewhat impede you-- but very, very seldom are you actually stopped from your weight-loss goals by genetics. In fact, pretty much never will you actually be unable to have a beautiful body; aside from the rare and unfortunate cases of physical deformity (and even sometimes people of exceptional will-power can overcome that)-- anyone can be beautiful if they put consistent effort into their diet and workout routine.

Last notable myth: You can't lose 10 pounds in 10 days.

Yes you can! Your body regularly goes through well over a pound of food a day. The high-protein and low-carb diet forces your body to start burning fat instead of relying on a steady intake of food to meet its caloric needs; that's why it works. Generally, for most regular people, you can expect to see 1 pound of fat to be lost every day for the first 10 days.

It isn't a magic pill; of course, it's a diet, and any change to how you eat is going to seem unpleasant at first. But you may actually really like being on a high-protein low-carb diet. You'll definitely like the results!

10 pounds in 10 days is totally possible. Chances are you've actually met someone who has done this without you even knowing that they have!

Chapter 6 – High Fat, Low Carbohydrate Slow Cooker Chicken Recipes

Chicken Chili Soup

Cooking Time: 6 Hours

Prep Time: 5 Minutes

Total Time: 6 Hours 5 Minutes

Serving Size: 1 ½ Cups

Nutritional Information

Protein: 41 Grams	Fat: 21 Grams	Carbohydrates: 7 Grams	Fiber: 2 Grams

Ingredients

- 8 Boneless Chicken Thighs
- 8 Slices Bacon
- 1 Pepper
- 1 Onion
- 2 Tbsp. Unsalted Butter
- 1 Tbsp. Thyme
- 1 tsp. Pepper
- 1 tsp. Salt
- 1 Tbsp. Minced Garlic

- 3 Tbsp. Lemon Juice
- 1 Tbsp. Coconut Flour
- 1 C. Chicken Stock
- ¼ C. Unsweetened Coconut Milk
- 3 Tbsp. Tomato Paste

Directions:

First, put the butter on the center of the crockpot and then thinly slice the onions and the peppers. Distribute the onions and peppers on the bottom of the crockpot and place in the chicken thighs evenly. Chop the eight slices of bacon and sprinkle them over the chicken. Add the seasonings, liquids, and tomato paste.

Cook everything on low for six hours. Breakup the chicken before serving; this should be easy as it is very tender. You can top it with sour cream and cheese if you'd like.

Buffalo Chicken

Cooking Time: 6 Hours

Prep Time: 5 Minutes

Total Time: 6 Hours 5 Minutes

Serving Size: 1 Cup

Nutritional Information

Protein: 52 Grams	Fat: 8 Grams	Carbohydrates: 1 Grams	Fiber: 0 Grams

Ingredients

- 3 Tbsp. Butter
- 1 Bottle Hot Sauce
- 6 Frozen Chicken Breasts
- ½ Pack Hidden Valley Ranch Seasoning

Directions

First, put the chicken in the crockpot and pour the hot sauce over the chicken. Then sprinkle the ranch seasoning over thetop. Cover it and cook it on low for six hours. Then shred the chicken and add the butter. Cook it for another hour on low.

Jerk Chicken

Cook Time: 6 Hours

Prep Time: 15 Minutes

Total Time: 6 Hours 15 Minutes

Serving Size: ½ Cup

Nutritional Information:

Protein: 18.9 Grams	Fat: 6.4 Grams	Carbohydrates: 1.8 Grams	Fiber: 0.2 Grams

Ingredients:

- 1 ½ lbs. Boneless Chicken Thighs
- 1 ½ Bone-In chicken Breasts
- ¼ C. Lime Juice
- 4 Garlic Cloves
- 2 Tbsp. Thyme
- 1 Tbsp. Fresh Ginger, Minced
- 1 Tbsp. Dark Brown Sugar
- 2 tsp. Allspice Berries
- 4 Scallions
- 3 Habanero Peppers, seeded
- 1 ½ tsp. Salt
- 2 Tbsp. White Vinegar
- 1 Red Pepper
- Salt
- Pepper

Directions:

Put all of the chicken in the crockpot. Then blend together the other ingredients in a blender until smooth. Pour this over the chicken and cook for six hours. Then shred the chicken before serving.

Thai Green Curry Chicken

Cook Time: 4 Hours 30 Minutes

Prep Time: 15 Minutes

Total Time: 4 Hours 45 Minutes

Serving Size: 1 Cup

Nutritional Information:

Protein: 35.5 Grams	Fat: 10.5 Grams	Carbohydrates: 5.9 Grams	Fiber: 1.5 Grams

Ingredients

- 1 ½ Cans Light Coconut Milk
- 3 Tbsp. Green Curry Paste
- 4 Garlic Cloves
- 3 Tbsp. Brown Sugar
- 2 ½ lbs. Chicken Breast, Cut Into Chunks
- 1 Bag Stir Fry Vegetables
- 1 Red Onions
- 1 Can Mini Corn
- 2 Tbsp. Cornstarch

Directions:

Whisk together the coconut milk, curry paste, garlic cloves, and brown sugar. Add the chicken, baby corn, onion, and vegetables. Then cook for four hours on low. After the cooking is finished, whisk together the cornstarch and add 2 tablespoons of water. Cook everything for another thirty minutes or until the curry is thickened.

Chapter 7 – High Fat, Low Carbohydrate Turkey Recipes

Turkey Herb Roast

Cook Time: 6 Hours on High, 10 Hours on Low

Prep Time: 5 Minutes

Total Time: 6 hours 5 Minutes on High, 10 Hours 5 Minutes on Low

Serving Size: 2 Cups

Nutritional Information:

Protein: 77.1 Grams	Fat: 41 Grams	Carbohydrates: 2.1 Grams	Fiber: 0.2 Grams

Ingredients:

- ½ Cup Cream Cheese
- 1/3 tsp. Garlic Powder
- 1/3 tsp. Dried Thyme
- 3 lbs. Turkey Breast
- 2 ½ Tbsp. Butter
- 1 Tbsp. Parsley
- 1 1/3 Tbsp. Soy Sauce
- ½ tsp. Sage
- ½ tsp. Basil

- ½ tsp. Pepper

Directions:

Mix all the ingredients together in a bowl and brush it over the turkey breast. Place the breast and remaining ingredients in the slow cooker and cook for ten hours on low or six hours on high.

Turkey Mercedes

Cook Time: 8 Hours on High

Prep Time: 15 Minutes

Total Time: 8 Hour and 15 Minutes

Serving Size: 1 Turkey

Nutritional Information:

Protein: 74.5 Grams	Fat: 25.6 Grams	Carbohydrates: 8.9 Grams	Fiber: 0.6 Grams

Ingredients:

- 3 Garlic Cloves
- 1 Tbsp. Pepper
- 1 Tbsp. Cumin
- 1 Tbsp. Oregano

- 2 Tbsp. Salt
- 2 C. Lemon Juice
- 1 C. White Wine
- ½ Can Frozen Orange Juice
- 1 (16 lbs.) Turkey

Directions:

Place turkey in the crockpot and mix ingredients together in a food process to blend gently. Put everything in the crockpot and cook on high for eight hours. Check for doneness.

Navy Style Turkey

Cook Time: 8 Hours on High

Prep Time: 15 Minutes

Total Time: 8 Hours and 15 Minutes

Serving Size: 1 Turkey

Nutritional Information:

Protein: 111.3 Grams	Fat: 53.7 Grams	Carbohydrates: 7.3 Grams	Fiber: 1.5 Grams

Ingredients:

- 1 (18lb.) Turkey
- 1 ¼ C. Butter
- 1 lb. Baby Carrots
- 2 Onions
- 3 Stalks Celery
- 1 Garlic Clove
- 3 Tbsp. Thyme
- 3 Tbsp. Sage
- 2 Bay Leaves
- 1 Bottle Chardonnay
- Salt and Pepper

Directions:

Remove the neck and giblet from the turkey and rinse the bird, then pat it dry. Place it in the crockpot and put the butter under the turkey's skin and secure it with toothpicks. Then mix together the onions, carrots, celery, garlic cloves, sage, thyme, bay leaves, salt, and pepper. Stuff the turkey with as much of this as possible. Pour the bottle of Chardonnay over the bird and roast for 8 hours on high.

Flavorful Turkey

Cook Time: 8 Hours on High

Prep Time: 15 Minutes

Total Time: 8 Hours and 15 Minutes

Serving Size: 1 Turkey

Nutritional Information:

| Protein: 91.3 Grams | Fat: 40.3 Grams | Carbohydrates: 6.1 Grams | Fiber: 1.3 Grams |

Ingredients:

- ½ C. Butter
- 1 (12 lb.) Turkey
- 1 Tbsp. Olive Oil
- 2 Apples
- 1 Onion
- ½ Garlic head
- 1 lb. Celery
- 1 Tbsp. Poultry Seasoning

Directions:

Rub the skin of the bird with the olive oil and stuff it with the remaining ingredients, except the butter. Place the butter under the skin and cook on high for eight hours, or until the bird reads 180°F.

Chapter 8 - High Fat, Low Carbohydrate Beef Recipes

Beef Pot Roast I

Cook Time: 6 Hours and 30 Minutes

Prep Time: 20 Minutes

Total Time: 6 Hours and 20 Minutes

Serving Size: 2 Cups

Nutritional Information:

Protein: 54.5 Grams	Fat: 57.3 Grams	Carbohydrates: 7.5 Grams	Fiber: 1.5 Grams

Ingredients:

- 1 5 lb. Beef Pot Roast
- Salt and Pepper
- 1 Tbsp. Flour
- 2 Tbsp. Olive Oil
- 8 Ounces Mushrooms, sliced
- 1 Onion
- 2 Garlic Cloves, minced
- 1 Tbsp. Butter
- 1 ½ Tbsp. Flour

- 1 Tbsp. Tomato Paste
- 2 ½ C. Chicken Broth
- 3 Carrots
- 2 Celery Stalks
- 1 Sprig Rosemary
- 2 Sprigs Thyme

Directions:

Rinse and pat dry the roast and sprinkle with salt and pepper. Sprinkle the flour over the roast until it's well coated and shake off any excess. Heat the vegetables in a skillet until they're hot, and then sear the roast on both sides for five to six minutes until it's well browned. Remove the meat from the skillet and set it aside.

Add the onion, garlic, and mushrooms and cook for five minutes with each addition. Then add 1 ½ Tbsp. flour and cook for another minute. Add the tomato paste and cook for another minute. Then add the chicken stock and stir to combine. Place the carrots and celery in the slow cooker. Put the roast over the vegetables and add the rosemary and thyme. Then add the onion and mushroom and cover the slow cooker. Cook on high for five to six hours.

Mexican Style Meat

Cook Time: 8 Hours

Prep Time: 30 Minutes

Total Time: 8 Hours and 30 Minutes

Serving Size: 2 Cups

Nutritional Information:

Protein: 18.4 Grams	Fat: 19.1 Grams	Carbohydrates: 3.3 Grams	Fiber: 0.7 Grams

Ingredients:

- 1 (4 lb.) Chuck Roast
- 1 tsp. Salt
- 1 tsp. Pepper
- 2 Tbsp. Olive Oil
- 1 Onion
- 1 ¼ C. Green Chile Pepper, diced
- 1 tsp. Chili Powder
- 1 tsp. Ground Cayenne
- 1 5oz. Bottle Hot Pepper Sauce
- 1 tsp. Garlic Powder

Directions:

Trim the roast of excess fat and season with salt and pepper. Heat the olive oil in a skillet and sear the beef. Transfer the roast to the slow cooker and top it with chopped onion. Season the roast with the rest of the ingredients and cook on high for six hours.Then reduce it to low and cook for another two to four hours.

Beef Pot Roast II

Cook Time: 11 Hours

Prep Time: 15 Minutes

Total Time: 11Hours and 15 Minutes

Serving Size: 2 Cups

Nutritional Information:

Protein: 45.6 Grams	Fat: 23.7 Grams	Carbohydrates: 4.9 Grams	Fiber: 0.1 Grams

Ingredients:

- 2 10.75oz. Cans Condensed Cream of Mushroom Soup
- 1oz. Package of Dry Onion Soup Mix
- 1 ¼ C. water
- 5 ½ lb. Roast

Directions:

Mix the cream of mushroom soup, dry onion soup mix and water in the crockpot. Then place the roast in and coat with the soup mixture. Cook on high for three to four hours and low for eight to nine hours.

Roast Beef

Cook Time: 8 Hours

Prep Time: 15 Minutes

Total Time: 8 Hours and 15 Minutes

Serving Size: 2 Cups

Nutritional Information:

Protein: 35.3 Grams	Fat: 16.1 Grams	Carbohydrates: 3.3 Grams	Fiber: 0 Grams

Ingredients:

- 3 lb. Rump Roast
- 1 10.75oz. Can Condensed Cream of Mushroom Soup
- 1 10.75 oz. can Condensed Beef Broth

Directions:

Place all ingredients in the slow cooker and cook for eight hours on low.

Chapter 9 - High Fat, Low Carbohydrate Pork Recipes

Asian Style Ribs

Cook Time: 17 Hours

Prep Time: 10 Minutes

Total Time: 17 Hours and 10 Minutes

Serving Size: 2 Cups

Nutritional Information:

Protein: 48.4 Grams	Fat: 44 Grams	Carbohydrates: 13.9 Grams	Fiber: 0.5 Grams

Ingredients:

- ¼ C. Brown Sugar
- 1 C. Soy Sauce
- ¼ C. Sesame Oil
- 2 Tbsp. Olive Oil
- 2 Tbsp. Rice Vinegar
- 2 Tbsp. Lime Juice
- 2 Tbsp. Minced Garlic
- 2 Tbsp. Ginger
- 1 tsp. Sriracha Hot Pepper Sauce

- 12 Pork Ribs

Directions:

Stir together the brown sugar up to the Sriracha sauce and place it in the crock pot. Then add the ribs, cover and refrigerate for at least eight hours or overnight. Then drain the marinade and discard. Cook for nine hours on low. Drain the meat and shred it using two forks.

Spicy Green Chili Pork

Cook Time: 8 Hours

Prep Time: 10 Minutes

Total Time: 8 Hours and 10 Minutes

Serving Size: 2 Cups

Nutritional Information:

Protein: 15.9 Grams	Fat: 8.4 Grams	Carbohydrates: 5.4 Grams	Fiber: 0.4 Grams

Ingredients:

- 1 Onion
- Salt and Pepper
- 2 ½ Lb. Pork Shoulder Roast

- 1 16 oz. Jar Green Salsa
- ½ C. Chopped Cilantro, Fresh
- 2 Serrano Chile Peppers

Directions:

Layer the onions in the bottom of the slow cooker and season the pork shoulder with salt and pepper. Place the pork shoulder on top of the onions and pour the green salsa over top. Sprinkle the cilantro over the pork and drop the peppers into the slow cooker.

Cook on low until the meat is falling apart easily, about eight hours. Remove the pork to a cutting board and discard half the remaining liquid in the crock pot. Then discard the onions and peppers. Shred the pork and mix it with the reserved liquid before serving.

Lancaster County Pork and Sauerkraut

Cook Time: 6 Hours

Prep Time: 20 Minutes

Total Time: 6 Hours and 20 Minutes

Serving Size: 2 Cups

Nutritional Information:

Protein: 36.8 Grams	Fat: 8.5 Grams	Carbohydrates: 3.5 Grams	Fiber: 2.2 Grams

Ingredients:

- 1 4lb. Pork Loin Roast
- 1 tsp. Caraway Seeds
- Salt and Pepper
- 2 C. Sauerkraut

Directions:

Cut the loin if you need to in order to fit it into the slow cooker. Season it with the caraway seeds, salt and pepper to your taste. Then pour the sauerkraut over the roast and cook on high for one hour. Then cook on low for five to six hours. The temperature should be 145 degrees F.

Pork Roast with Sauerkraut and Kielbasa

Cook Time: 6 Hours

Prep Time: 25 Minutes

Total Time: 6 Hours and 25 Minutes

Serving Size: 2 Cups

Nutritional Information:

Protein: 14.8 Grams	Fat: 15.7 Grams	Carbohydrates: 7.6 Grams	Fiber: 4 Grams

Ingredients:

- 1 2lb. Pork Loin Roast, Boneless
- 2 Tbsp. Olive Oil
- 2 Sprigs Thyme Leaves
- Salt and Pepper
- 4 lbs. Sauerkraut
- 1 lb. Kielbasa, cut in 3 in. pieces

Directions:

Preheat your broiler and place the roast on a roasting pan. Then brush the roast with olive oil, sprinkle it with the thyme leaves, and season it with the salt and pepper. Place it in the broiler for ten minutes or until it's browned in several places. Then put the sauerkraut in the slow cooker and arrange the kielbasa pieces around the edges. Put the roast in the center and cover it with the sauerkraut using a fork. Cook it on high for six hours or until it's tender.

Conclusion

As a recap, high-protein and low-carb diets work by forcing your body to source its energy from protein; which is much less of an efficient way for extracting energy than the fat that's already on or in your body. So a high-protein low-carb diet will tend to make you burn fat-weight and build muscle.

There are three primary, fundamental, inescapable rules to weight loss. Eat less, move more, and keep breathing.

This diet is a trick to enhance that. It gives you energy to move and also increases the effectiveness of how you lose weight through cellular respiration and breathing out carbon dioxide.

We went over the history of our species, and covered how our ancestors probably survived on diets not too dissimilar from these ones. So, while there are some health-risks to keep in mind, you can know for certain that you're able to survive on a diet like this. Though it's recommended that you only use these diets to burn up fat and lose body-fat percentage points.

Then we covered some of the myths surrounding weight-loss. Stop blaming your genetics and put some effort in! People can still get fat from 'fat free' diets! Calories aren't absolutely everything you need to know; there's more to it than that! Ab workouts are to be taken lightly according to many body-builders! And yes; it's always going to take effort to change your physique for the better; there's no getting around that!

Hopefully this guide will be a good resource for you in your weight-loss goals, and can lead you on the quickest path to a better body and a happier life. It outlines the quickest way for you to safely lose weight in a proven way. The high-protein low-carb diet is the fastest way to train your body into burning fat, and the typical person can burn up to 10 pounds of fat in just 10 days. Odds are, you can too if you stick to this diet and moderately exercise.

Thank you for downloading our Ebook!

We hope you have enjoyed the reading.

Please Read our next Tips:

1. The Skinny Gut Diet: How to Lose up to 10 pounds in 30 days. 30-Day Skinny Gut Diet for Weight loss.

Made in the USA
Columbia, SC
08 July 2025